VEG IBS Relief
DIET COOKBOOK

50+ Easy-to-Make Delicious Low-FODMAP Recipes and 21-Day Meal Plan to Soothe Irritable Bowel Syndrome Symptoms

AMELIA BLYTHE

Copyright © 2024 by **Amelia Blythe**
All rights reserved.

No part of this book may be reproduced, distributed, or transmitted in any form or by any means, including photocopying, recording, or other electronic or mechanical methods, without the prior written permission of the publisher, except in the case of brief quotations embodied in critical reviews and certain other noncommercial uses permitted by copyright law.

OTHER BOOKS BY THE AUTHOR

- **VEGETARIAN ANTI-INFLAMMATORY DIET COOKBOOK FOR SENIORS**

- **VEGETARIAN IRON DEFICIENCY ANEMIA COOKBOOK**

- **VEGETARIAN LOW CHOLESTEROL DIET COOKBOOK FOR SENIORS**

- **VEGAN LOW-CHOLESTEROL DIET COOKBOOK FOR SENIORS**

- **THE PLANT BASED LOW-CHOLESTEROL DIET COOKBOOK FOR SENIORS**

TABLE OF CONTENTS

INTRODUCTION 7
CHAPTER 1 9
UNDERSTANDING IRRITABLE BOWEL SYNDROME (IBS) 9
    Causes of IBS 9
    Symptoms of IBS 9
    Risk Factors for IBS 10
    Types of IBS 10
    Treatment/Home Remedies 11
    Overview of the Low FODMAP Approach for IBS 11
CHAPTER 3 13
IBS-FRIENDLY VEGAN STAPLES 13
    Essential Low FODMAP Vegan Ingredients 13
    Common IBS Triggers and How to Avoid Them .. 15
    Stocking an IBS-Friendly Vegan Pantry 16
CHAPTER 4 17
BREAKFAST RECIPES 17
    Low-FODMAP Banana Blueberry Overnight Oats 17
    Ginger-Spiced Carrot Smoothie Bowl 19

Coconut Chia Pudding with Fresh Strawberries.. 21
Maple Cinnamon Quinoa Breakfast Bowl 22
Spinach Bell Pepper Tofu Scramble 23
Buckwheat Pancakes with Raspberries 25
Almond Butter and Banana Rice Cakes 27
Warm Oatmeal with Pumpkin Seeds and Kiwi....28
Zucchini and Sweet Potato Hash 29

CHAPTER 5 31

LUNCH RECIPES 31

Quinoa and Roasted Vegetable Salad 31
Zucchini Noodle Salad with Peanut Dressing 33
Sweet Potato and Spinach Buddha Bowl 35
Chickpea Salad Wraps 37
Mediterranean Rice Bowl 38
Lentil and Bell Pepper Stuffed Bell Peppers 39
Tofu and Spinach Stir-Fry with Rice Noodles 41
Carrot Ginger Soup with Coconut Milk 43
Tempeh and Roasted Veggie Grain Bowl 45
Cucumber Avocado Rice Sushi Rolls 47

CHAPTER 6 49

DINNER RECIPES 49

Stir-Fried Tofu with Zucchini and Carrots 49

Stuffed Sweet Potatoes with Spinach and Quinoa 51
Roasted Vegetable and Brown Rice Bowl 53
Tempeh Tacos with Cabbage and Lime Slaw 55
Coconut Curry with Bell Peppers and Carrots 57
Eggplant and Tomato Stew with Fresh Herbs 59
Baked Spaghetti Squash 61
Ginger and Turmeric Lentil Soup 63
Baked Polenta with Tomato Sauce 65

CHAPTER 7 67
SOUPS AND STEWS 67
Creamy Carrot Ginger Soup 67
Roasted Red Pepper Tomato Soup 69
Butternut Squash Sage Soup 71
Pumpkin Bell Pepper Stew 73
Zucchini and Corn Chowder 75
Sweet Potato and Coconut Milk Stew 77
Spinach Potato Dill Soup 78
Celeriac Parsnip Soup 79
Spinach and Quinoa Vegetable Soup 81

CHAPTER 8 83
SNACKS AND DESSERTS 83
Almond Butter Chia Energy Balls 83

Blueberry Chia Pudding Parfait 85
Lemon Coconut Energy Balls 86
Banana and Oatmeal Cookies 87
Cinnamon Roasted Pumpkin Seeds 89
Coconut Yogurt with Kiwi and Strawberries 90
Chocolate-Dipped Rice Cakes with Almonds 91
Peanut Butter Banana Nice Cream 93
Baked Carrot Chips with Paprika 94

CHAPTER 9 95
SMOOTHIES AND BEVERAGES 95

Peach and Ginger Smoothie 95
Blueberry and Coconut Water Smoothie 96
Pineapple and Ginger Green Smoothie................ 97
Strawberry and Mint Lemonade 98
Banana and Almond Milk Smoothie 99
Turmeric Golden Milk with Coconut Milk 100
Raspberry and Basil Infused Water 101
Carrot Ginger Juice 102

21-DAY MEAL PLAN 103
CONCLUSION 109

INTRODUCTION

Irritable Bowel Syndrome (IBS) is a common yet complex gastrointestinal disorder that affects *approximately 10-15%* of the global population. In the United States alone, it is estimated *that around 25 to 45 million people* suffer from IBS, with women being affected nearly twice as often as men.

Though it can appear at any age, IBS is most often diagnosed in individuals under the age of 50. Characterized by symptoms like *abdominal pain, bloating, constipation, diarrhea, and irregular bowel movements*, IBS can significantly impact daily life and wellbeing. Yet, despite its prevalence, there is no one-size-fits-all solution for managing it.

For those who follow a vegan diet, navigating IBS can feel challenging. Many traditional approaches to IBS management, such as the Low FODMAP diet, focus on removing certain fermentable carbohydrates that can trigger symptoms.

While effective, this approach can feel restrictive, particularly for vegans who rely on legumes, grains, and certain vegetables as primary protein and nutrient sources. However, with a thoughtful approach, it's entirely possible to create a vegan, IBS-friendly diet that's both nourishing and satisfying.

This cookbook is designed to bridge the gap, providing a practical resource for anyone looking to manage IBS symptoms on a vegan diet. From low-FODMAP staples to symptom-soothing recipes, you'll find accessible, nutrient-dense options to support digestive health and reduce IBS flare-ups.

Whether you're seeking long-term symptom relief or just a way to add more variety to your daily meals, this book offers practical, compassionate support to help you along your journey.

Let's get started on crafting meals that nourish, soothe, and support your health from the inside out.

CHAPTER 1

UNDERSTANDING IRRITABLE BOWEL SYNDROME (IBS)

Irritable Bowel Syndrome (IBS) is a functional gastrointestinal disorder that affects the large intestine, leading to a range of symptoms.

Causes of IBS

The exact cause of IBS remains unclear, but it is thought to involve multiple factors, including abnormal intestinal contractions, increased sensitivity to pain, disruptions in gut bacteria, and stress. Hormonal changes and certain foods can also trigger IBS symptoms.

Symptoms of IBS

The symptoms of IBS typically include abdominal pain, bloating, gas, cramping, and altered bowel habits such as diarrhea, constipation, or a combination of both. Symptoms vary from person to person and can range in severity, often impacting daily life and overall quality of life.

Risk Factors for IBS

The risk factors for IBS include a family history of the disorder, mental health issues like anxiety or depression, and early life stressors. It's more common in younger adults and in women, with hormonal fluctuations believed to play a role. Certain dietary choices and lifestyle factors, such as lack of sleep and high stress levels, can also exacerbate IBS.

Types of IBS

There are three primary **types of IBS** based on predominant symptoms:

1. **IBS-D (IBS with Diarrhea)**: Characterized by frequent, loose stools.

2. **IBS-C (IBS with Constipation)**: Associated with hard, infrequent stools.

3. **IBS-M (Mixed IBS)**: Includes both diarrhea and constipation episodes.

Treatment/Home Remedies

The treatment/home remedies for IBS often involve a combination of lifestyle changes, dietary adjustments, and stress management. Many people with IBS find symptom relief by following a *balanced diet, increasing fiber intake (especially soluble fiber), staying hydrated, and engaging in regular physical activity*.

Some home remedies, such as peppermint oil, ginger, and probiotics, have shown promise in alleviating symptoms. *Stress management techniques*—such as *yoga, meditation, and deep breathing exercises*—can help reduce IBS-related symptoms by lowering cortisol levels and promoting relaxation.

Overview of the Low FODMAP Approach for IBS

The Low FODMAP diet is a scientifically supported approach that aims to reduce the intake of certain types of fermentable carbohydrates known to trigger IBS symptoms.

FODMAP stands for *Fermentable Oligosaccharides, Disaccharides, Monosaccharides, and Polyols*—types of carbohydrates that can be poorly absorbed in the small intestine and lead to gas, bloating, and other digestive issues as they ferment in the colon.

The Low FODMAP approach consists of three phases:

1. **Elimination Phase**: All high-FODMAP foods are removed from the diet for a period, typically 2-6 weeks, to reduce symptoms.

2. **Reintroduction Phase**: High-FODMAP foods are gradually reintroduced one at a time to identify individual triggers.

3. **Personalization Phase**: After identifying tolerable FODMAPs, a balanced diet is customized to incorporate safe foods.

While effective, the Low FODMAP diet requires careful planning, as common plant-based foods like beans, certain vegetables, and grains are restricted in the elimination phase. However, low-FODMAP vegan-friendly options—like firm tofu, quinoa, and certain fruits and vegetables (e.g., zucchini, carrots, and bananas)—make it feasible to follow a plant-based Low FODMAP approach.

CHAPTER 3

IBS-FRIENDLY VEGAN STAPLES

Essential Low FODMAP Vegan Ingredients

Creating delicious and IBS-friendly vegan meals begins with choosing low FODMAP ingredients that don't aggravate the digestive system.

Key staples for a low FODMAP vegan diet include:

- **Proteins**: Firm tofu and tempeh are excellent low FODMAP sources of protein. Lentils and chickpeas are allowed in limited quantities if canned and well-rinsed, as this process reduces FODMAP content.

  Other options include nuts (such as almonds and walnuts) in small servings, as well as chia seeds and pumpkin seeds.

- **Grains and Carbohydrates**: Gluten-free grains like quinoa, rice, oats, and buckwheat are well-tolerated. Small amounts of sourdough spelt bread can also be suitable. These grains provide fiber without triggering symptoms.

- **Fruits**: Low FODMAP fruits, eaten in moderation, include bananas, blueberries, strawberries, oranges, and kiwis. These fruits are gentle on the digestive system while offering vitamins and antioxidants.

- **Vegetables**: Carrots, zucchini, bell peppers, spinach, and potatoes are all low FODMAP vegetables that are versatile and gentle on digestion. *Avoid high-FODMAP options like garlic and onions, which are common triggers.*

- **Dairy Substitutes**: Plant-based milk alternatives, like almond milk, coconut milk (from the carton), and lactose-free soy milk, are generally low FODMAP and good choices for those avoiding dairy.

- **Fats and Oils**: Olive oil, coconut oil, and small amounts of avocado are good fats that support gut health. Since fats can stimulate digestion, they should be used in moderation to avoid potential discomfort.

Common IBS Triggers and How to Avoid Them

Certain foods and ingredients are well-known triggers that can worsen symptoms. These include:

- **High-FODMAP Foods**: Ingredients like onions, garlic, cauliflower, mushrooms, and certain beans contain high FODMAPs that can lead to bloating and discomfort. Using alternatives, such *as garlic-infused oil instead of whole garlic,* can add flavor without the IBS triggers.

- **Insoluble Fiber**: High amounts of insoluble fiber, found in foods like *raw greens, cabbage, and whole grains*, can be hard to digest. Instead, focus on soluble fiber from *oats, chia seeds, and well-cooked vegetables*, which is gentler on the stomach.

- **Caffeine and Alcohol**: These can overstimulate the digestive system, leading to cramping and irritation. Herbal teas and low-caffeine beverages are better options, and limiting alcohol can help prevent flare-ups.

- **Spicy and High-Fat Foods**: Both of these can worsen IBS symptoms for some people. Mild seasonings, such as ginger, turmeric, and cinnamon, are flavorful alternatives to hot spices.

Stocking an IBS-Friendly Vegan Pantry

A well-organized, IBS-friendly vegan pantry makes meal preparation easier and helps you stick to a soothing diet. Here are some essentials:

- **Canned and Dried Goods**: Stock up on canned, low-FODMAP legumes, like chickpeas and lentils, as they're quick and easy sources of protein and fiber. Keep gluten-free grains like rice and oats, as well as low-FODMAP pasta options, on hand.

- **Flavor Enhancers**: Since garlic and onions are high FODMAP, garlic-infused oils, fresh herbs, ginger, and low-FODMAP spices like turmeric and basil can add flavor. Nutritional yeast is another IBS-friendly way to add a cheesy taste to dishes.

- **Vegan Dairy Alternatives**: Keep plant-based, low-FODMAP options like almond milk, coconut yogurt, and lactose-free soy milk. These provide creamy textures for cooking and baking without upsetting the stomach.

- **Gut-Friendly Snacks**: Keep simple, low-FODMAP snacks like rice cakes, pumpkin seeds, low-FODMAP fruits, and nut butters in small portions. These are easy to digest and can help manage hunger between meals.

CHAPTER 4

BREAKFAST RECIPES

Low-FODMAP Banana Blueberry Overnight Oats

Prep Time: 5 minutes
Chill Time: overnight soaking
Servings: 1

Ingredients:

- ½ cup rolled oats (gluten-free)
- ½ cup almond milk (unsweetened, or other low-FODMAP plant-based milk)
- ½ ripe banana, mashed
- ¼ cup fresh blueberries
- 1 tbsp chia seeds
- ½ tsp maple syrup (optional, for sweetness)
- ¼ tsp cinnamon (optional, for flavor)

Instructions:

1. In a mason jar or small bowl, combine the rolled oats, almond milk, mashed banana, chia seeds, and cinnamon.

2. Stir well until all ingredients are evenly mixed.

3. Top with fresh blueberries and a drizzle of maple syrup if desired.

4. Cover and refrigerate overnight (at least 6-8 hours).

5. In the morning, give the oats a good stir and enjoy directly from the jar or transfer to a bowl.

Nutritional Val. (per serving):

- **Calories**: ~290 kcal
- **Protein**: 6g
- **Carbohydrates**: 50g
- **Fiber**: 8g
- **Sugars**: 10g
- **Fat**: 7g

Ginger-Spiced Carrot Smoothie Bowl

Prep Time: 10 minutes
Cook Time: None
Servings: 1

Ingredients:

- 1 medium carrot, peeled and chopped (steamed and cooled for a smoother texture)
- ½ ripe banana
- ½ cup almond milk (unsweetened, or another low-FODMAP plant-based milk)
- ¼ tsp fresh grated ginger (or 1/8 tsp ground ginger)
- ½ tsp cinnamon
- 1 tbsp chia seeds (optional, for thickness and added fiber)
- Toppings: 1 tbsp pumpkin seeds, ¼ cup blueberries, shredded coconut (optional)

Instructions:

1. In a blender, combine the carrot, banana, almond milk, ginger, and cinnamon. Add chia seeds if you want a thicker consistency.
2. Blend until smooth and creamy.
3. Pour into a bowl and top with pumpkin seeds, blueberries, and a sprinkle of shredded coconut if desired.
4. Serve immediately and enjoy.

Nutritional Values (per serving):

- **Calories**: ~200 kcal
- **Protein**: 4g
- **Carbohydrates**: 36g
- **Fiber**: 7g
- **Sugars**: 15g
- **Fat**: 6g

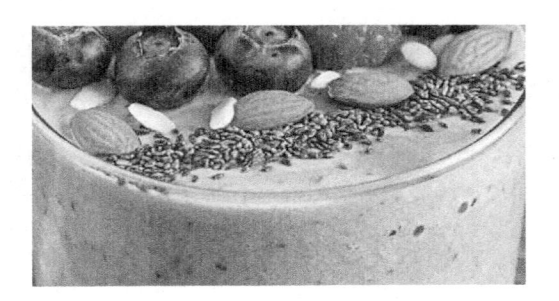

Coconut Chia Pudding with Fresh Strawberries

Prep Time: 5 minutes

Servings: 1

Nutritional Val. (per serving): Calories: ~180 kcal; Protein: 4g Carbs: 20g; Fiber: 8g; Fat: 8g

Ingredients:

- ½ cup almond milk or carton coconut milk (low-FODMAP variety)
- 2 tbsp chia seeds
- ½ tsp vanilla extract (optional)
- 1 tsp maple syrup (optional)
- ¼ cup fresh strawberries, sliced

Instructions:

1. In a small bowl or jar, whisk together the almond or coconut milk, chia seeds, vanilla extract, and maple syrup.
2. Stir well to ensure the chia seeds are evenly distributed.
3. Cover and refrigerate for at least 2 hours or overnight, until the chia seeds have absorbed the liquid and formed a gel-like consistency.
4. Before serving, top with fresh strawberry slices.
5. Enjoy chilled.

Maple Cinnamon Quinoa Breakfast Bowl

Prep Time: 5 minutes
Cook Time: 15 minutes
Servings: 2

Nutritional Val (per serving):
Calories: ~220 kcal; Protein: 6g
Carbs: 36g; Fiber: 5g; Fat: 5g

Ingredients:
- ½ cup quinoa, rinsed
- 1 cup almond milk
- 1 tbsp maple syrup
- ¼ tsp ground cinnamon
- ¼ cup fresh blueberries
- 1 tbsp chia seeds (optional)

Instructions:
1. In a small saucepan, combine the rinsed quinoa and almond milk. Bring to a boil over medium heat.
2. Reduce the heat to low, cover, and simmer for about 15 minutes, or until the quinoa is cooked and the liquid is absorbed.
3. Stir in the maple syrup and cinnamon.
4. Divide the quinoa into bowls and top with fresh blueberries and chia seeds, if desired.
5. Serve warm.

Spinach Bell Pepper Tofu Scramble

Prep Time: 10 minutes
Cook Time: 10 minutes
Servings: 2

Ingredients:

- 1 block (200g) firm tofu, drained and crumbled
- 1 tbsp olive oil
- 1 cup fresh spinach, chopped
- ½ red bell pepper, diced
- ¼ tsp turmeric powder
- ¼ tsp cumin powder
- Salt and pepper to taste
- Fresh parsley or chives, for garnish (optional)

Instructions:

1. In a skillet, heat olive oil over medium heat.
2. Add the diced red bell pepper and cook for 2-3 minutes, until softened.

3. Add the crumbled tofu to the skillet, along with the turmeric and cumin. Stir well to combine.

4. Cook the tofu for 3-4 minutes, stirring occasionally until lightly browned.

5. Add the chopped spinach and cook for another 1-2 minutes, until wilted.

6. Season with salt and pepper to taste.

7. Serve warm, garnished with fresh parsley or chives if desired.

Nutritional Values (per serving):

- **Calories**: ~170 kcal
- **Protein**: 12g
- **Carbohydrates**: 7g
- **Fiber**: 2g
- **Sugars**: 2g
- **Fat**: 11g

Buckwheat Pancakes with Raspberries

Prep Time: 10 minutes
Cook Time: 10 minutes
Servings: 4 small pancakes (2 servings)

Ingredients:

- ½ cup buckwheat flour
- ½ cup almond milk (unsweetened, or another low-FODMAP plant-based milk)
- 1 tbsp maple syrup (optional, for sweetness)
- ½ tsp baking powder
- ¼ tsp vanilla extract (optional)
- Cooking spray or 1 tsp coconut oil, for greasing
- ¼ cup fresh raspberries (for topping)

Instructions:

1. In a mixing bowl, whisk together the buckwheat flour, almond milk, baking powder, maple syrup, and vanilla extract until smooth.

2. Heat a non-stick skillet over medium heat and lightly grease with cooking spray or coconut oil.

3. Pour a small amount of batter into the skillet to form a pancake. Cook for 2-3 minutes, or until bubbles form on the surface. Flip and cook for another 1-2 minutes on the other side.

4. Repeat with the remaining batter.

5. Serve pancakes topped with fresh raspberries.

Nutritional Values (per serving):
- **Calories**: ~190 kcal
- **Protein**: 5g
- **Carbohydrates**: 30g
- **Fiber**: 4g
- **Sugars**: 5g
- **Fat**: 4g

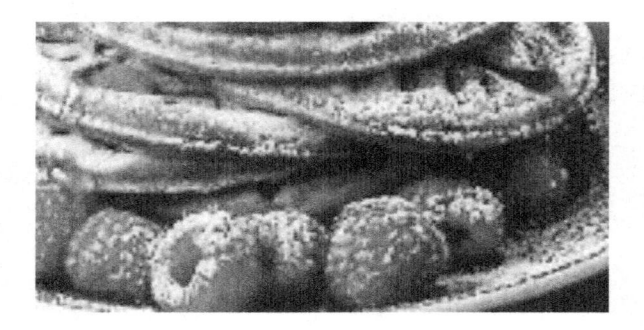

Almond Butter and Banana Rice Cakes

Prep Time: 5 minutes
Cook Time: None
Servings: 1

Ingredients:

- 2 plain rice cakes (unsalted)
- 1 tbsp almond butter (smooth, without added sugars or oils)
- ½ ripe banana, sliced
- ¼ tsp cinnamon (optional, for extra flavor)

Instructions:

1. Spread the almond butter evenly over each rice cake.
2. Top with banana slices and sprinkle with a little cinnamon, if desired.
3. Serve immediately.

Nutritional Values (per serving):

- **Calories**: ~180 kcal; **Protein**: 4g
- **Carbs**: 28g; **Fiber**: 3g
- **Fat**: 7g

Warm Oatmeal with Pumpkin Seeds and Kiwi

Prep Time: 5 minutes
Cook Time: 5 minutes
Servings: 1

Ingredients:

- ½ cup rolled oats (gluten-free)
- 1 cup water or almond milk (unsweetened, or another low-FODMAP plant-based milk)
- ½ tsp cinnamon
- 1 kiwi, peeled and sliced
- 1 tbsp pumpkin seeds
- 1 tsp maple syrup (optional, for sweetness)

Instructions:

1. In a small saucepan, bring the water or almond milk to a boil. Add the oats and cinnamon.

2. Reduce the heat and simmer, stirring occasionally, for about 5 minutes or until the oats are tender and the liquid is absorbed.

3. Transfer the oatmeal to a bowl and top with sliced kiwi, pumpkin seeds, and a drizzle of maple syrup if desired.

4. Serve warm.

Zucchini and Sweet Potato Hash

Prep Time: 10 minutes
Cook Time: 15 minutes
Servings: 2

Ingredients:

- 1 medium zucchini, diced
- 1 medium sweet potato, peeled and diced
- 1 tbsp olive oil
- ½ red bell pepper, diced
- ¼ tsp paprika
- Salt and pepper to taste
- Fresh parsley or chives, for garnish (optional)

Instructions:

1. In a large skillet, heat the olive oil over medium heat.

2. Add the diced sweet potato and cook for 8-10 minutes, stirring occasionally, until it begins to soften and brown.

3. Add the zucchini, red bell pepper, paprika, salt, and pepper. Continue to cook for another 5-7 minutes, or until the zucchini is tender and the sweet potato is fully cooked.

4. Garnish with fresh parsley or chives if desired, and serve warm.

Nutritional Values (per serving):
- **Calories**: ~160 kcal
- **Protein**: 2g
- **Carbohydrates**: 20g
- **Fiber**: 5g
- **Sugars**: 5g
- **Fat**: 8g

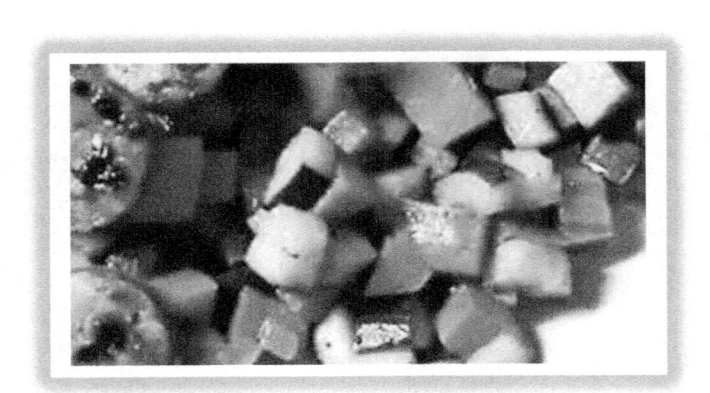

CHAPTER 5

LUNCH RECIPES

Quinoa and Roasted Vegetable Salad

Prep Time: 10 minutes
Cook Time: 25 minutes
Servings: 2

Ingredients:

- ½ cup quinoa, rinsed
- 1 cup water
- 1 small zucchini, diced
- 1 red bell pepper, diced
- 1 medium carrot, sliced
- 1 tbsp olive oil
- Salt and pepper, to taste
- 1 tbsp fresh parsley, chopped (optional)
- 1 tbsp pumpkin seeds (optional, for crunch)

Instructions:

1. Preheat the oven to 400°F (200°C). Line a baking sheet with parchment paper.

2. Place the zucchini, red bell pepper, and carrot on the baking sheet. Drizzle with olive oil, season with salt and pepper, and toss to coat. Roast for 20-25 minutes, stirring halfway, until the vegetables are tender and slightly browned.

3. Meanwhile, in a small pot, bring water to a boil, add the quinoa, and reduce heat to low. Cover and simmer for about 15 minutes or until the water is absorbed. Remove from heat and let it sit for 5 minutes, then fluff with a fork.

4. In a mixing bowl, combine the cooked quinoa and roasted vegetables. Toss gently to combine.

5. Sprinkle with fresh parsley and pumpkin seeds, if desired, before serving.

Nutritional Values (per serving):

- **Calories**: ~250 kcal; **Protein**: 7g
- **Carbohydrates**: 34g; **Fiber**: 6g
- **Sugars**: 6g
- **Fat**: 10g

Zucchini Noodle Salad with Peanut Dressing

Prep Time: 15 minutes
Servings: 2

Ingredients:

- 2 medium zucchinis, spiralized into noodles
- 1 medium carrot, julienned or grated
- ½ red bell pepper, thinly sliced
- 1 tbsp fresh cilantro, chopped (optional)

For the Peanut Dressing:

- 1 tbsp natural peanut butter (smooth, without added sugars)
- 1 tbsp tamari or soy sauce (low sodium)
- 1 tsp maple syrup
- 1 tbsp lime juice
- 1-2 tbsp water (to thin as needed)

Instructions:

1. In a small bowl, whisk together the peanut butter, tamari, maple syrup, lime juice, and water. Adjust the consistency by adding more water if needed.

2. In a large bowl, combine the zucchini noodles, carrot, and red bell pepper.

3. Pour the peanut dressing over the vegetables and toss gently to coat.

4. Garnish with fresh cilantro if desired, and serve immediately.

Nutritional Val (per serving):

- **Calories**: ~180 kcal
- **Protein**: 6g
- **Carbohydrates**: 22g
- **Fiber**: 5g
- **Sugars**: 8g
- **Fat**: 8g

Sweet Potato and Spinach Buddha Bowl

Prep Time: 10 minutes
Cook Time: 20 minutes
Servings: 2

Ingredients:

- 1 medium sweet potato, peeled and diced
- 1 tbsp olive oil
- Salt and pepper, to taste
- 1 cup fresh spinach, chopped
- ½ cup cooked quinoa or brown rice
- ¼ avocado, sliced (optional for creaminess)
- 1 tbsp pumpkin seeds or sunflower seeds (optional, for added texture)

For the Dressing:

- 1 tbsp tahini
- 1 tbsp lemon juice
- 1 tsp maple syrup
- 1-2 tbsp water (to thin as needed)

Instructions:

1. Preheat the oven to 400°F (200°C). Line a baking sheet with parchment paper.

2. Place the diced sweet potato on the baking sheet, drizzle with olive oil, and season with salt and pepper. Toss to coat, then roast for 20 minutes, stirring halfway through, until the sweet potato is tender.

3. Meanwhile, in a small bowl, whisk together the tahini, lemon juice, maple syrup, and water. Adjust consistency by adding more water if needed.

4. In serving bowls, add a base of cooked quinoa or brown rice. Layer with roasted sweet potato, fresh spinach, and avocado slices.

5. Drizzle with the tahini dressing and sprinkle with pumpkin or sunflower seeds, if desired.

6. Serve immediately.

Nutritional Values (per serving):

- **Calories**: ~300 kcal; **Protein**: 7g
- **Carbohydrates**: 38g
- **Fiber**: 8g; **Sugars**: 6g
- **Fat**: 12g

Chickpea Salad Wraps

Prep Time: 10 minutes
Servings: 2

Ingredients:

- ½ cup canned chickpeas, drained, rinsed, and mashed slightly (use a small serving to stay low-FODMAP)
- 1 tbsp tahini
- 1 tbsp lemon juice
- ½ tsp Dijon mustard
- Salt and pepper, to taste
- 1 small carrot, grated
- 1 celery stalk, finely chopped
- 1-2 lettuce leaves or low-FODMAP tortilla wrap (e.g., gluten-free wrap)

Instructions:

1. In a mixing bowl, combine the chickpeas, tahini, lemon juice, and Dijon mustard. Season with salt and pepper and mix until well combined.

2. Stir in the grated carrot and chopped celery.

3. Lay out the lettuce leaves or wrap, and spoon the chickpea mixture onto it.

4. Roll up and serve immediately.

Mediterranean Rice Bowl

Prep Time: 10 minutes
Cook Time: 15 minutes
Servings: 2

Nutritional Val (per serving):
Calories: ~220 kcal; Protein: 4g
Carbs: 32g; Fiber: 4g; Fat: 10g

Ingredients:

- 1 cup cooked rice (white or brown, according to preference)
- ½ cup diced cucumber
- ¼ cup cherry tomatoes, halved
- ¼ cup black or green olives, pitted and sliced
- 1 tbsp extra-virgin olive oil
- 1 tbsp lemon juice
- Salt and pepper, to taste
- Fresh basil or parsley for garnish (optional)

Instructions:

1. In a bowl, combine the cooked rice, cucumber, cherry tomatoes, and olives.

2. Drizzle with olive oil and lemon juice, then season with salt and pepper to taste.

3. Toss gently to combine, and garnish with fresh basil or parsley if desired.

4. Serve warm or chilled.

Lentil and Bell Pepper Stuffed Bell Peppers

Prep Time: 15 minutes
Cook Time: 25 minutes
Servings: 2

Ingredients:

- 2 large bell peppers (any color)
- ½ cup canned lentils, rinsed and drained (or cooked lentils)
- ½ cup cooked quinoa or rice
- ½ cup diced tomatoes (fresh or canned, no added onion or garlic)
- 1 tsp olive oil
- ¼ tsp dried basil
- Salt and pepper, to taste
- Fresh parsley, for garnish (optional)

Instructions:

1. Preheat the oven to 375°F (190°C).

2. Cut the tops off the bell peppers and remove the seeds and membranes.

3. In a bowl, mix the lentils, cooked quinoa or rice, diced tomatoes, olive oil, basil, salt, and pepper.

4. Stuff the bell peppers with the lentil mixture and place them in a baking dish.

5. Cover with foil and bake for 20-25 minutes, until the peppers are tender.

6. Garnish with fresh parsley, if desired, and serve warm.

Nutritional Val (per serving):
- **Calories**: ~200 kcal; **Protein**: 8g
- **Carbohydrates**: 35g
- **Fiber**: 8g
- **Sugars**: 7g
- **Fat**: 4g

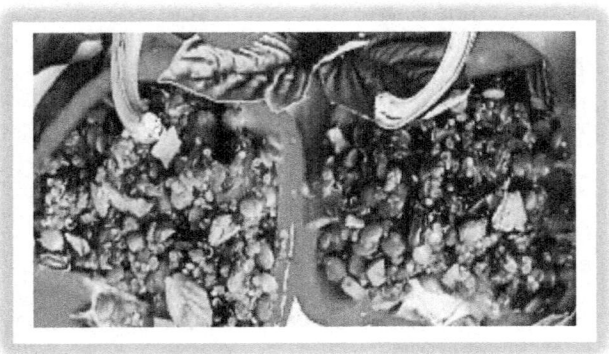

Tofu and Spinach Stir-Fry with Rice Noodles

Prep Time: 10 minutes
Cook Time: 15 minutes
Servings: 2

Ingredients:

- 4 oz rice noodles
- 1 tbsp sesame oil (or other neutral oil)
- ½ cup firm tofu, cubed
- 1 cup fresh spinach
- ½ red bell pepper, sliced
- 1 medium carrot, julienned
- 1 tbsp tamari or soy sauce (low sodium)
- 1 tbsp lime juice
- Salt and pepper, to taste
- Fresh cilantro, for garnish (optional)

Instructions:

1. Cook the rice noodles according to the package instructions. Drain and set aside.

2. In a large skillet or wok, heat sesame oil over medium heat. Add tofu cubes and cook for 4-5 minutes, until golden and crispy on all sides.

3. Add the red bell pepper and carrot to the skillet and stir-fry for 3-4 minutes, until slightly softened.

4. Add the spinach and cook until wilted, about 1-2 minutes.

5. Add the cooked noodles, tamari, and lime juice, and toss everything together. Season with salt and pepper to taste.

6. Garnish with fresh cilantro if desired and serve warm.

Nutritional Values (per serving):

- **Calories**: ~300 kcal
- **Protein**: 10g
- **Carbohydrates**: 42g
- **Fiber**: 5g
- **Sugars**: 4g
- **Fat**: 10g

Carrot Ginger Soup with Coconut Milk

Prep Time: 10 minutes
Cook Time: 20 minutes
Servings: 2

Ingredients:

- 1 tbsp olive oil
- 4 large carrots, peeled and sliced
- 1 tsp fresh ginger, grated (or ½ tsp ground ginger)
- 2 cups low-sodium vegetable broth
- ½ cup canned coconut milk (full-fat or light)
- Salt and pepper, to taste
- Fresh parsley, for garnish (optional)

Instructions:

1. In a medium pot, heat the olive oil over medium heat. Add the sliced carrots and grated ginger, and sauté for 5 minutes, until the carrots begin to soften.

2. Pour in the vegetable broth and bring to a boil. Reduce heat and let simmer for 15 minutes, or until the carrots are tender.

3. Remove the pot from heat. Using an immersion blender (or carefully transferring to a blender), blend the soup until smooth.

4. Stir in the coconut milk and season with salt and pepper to taste.

5. Serve warm, garnished with fresh parsley if desired.

Nutritional Values (per serving):

- **Calories**: ~180 kcal
- **Protein**: 2g
- **Carbohydrates**: 20g
- **Fiber**: 5g
- **Sugars**: 8g
- **Fat**: 12g

Tempeh and Roasted Veggie Grain Bowl

Prep Time: 10 minutes
Cook Time: 25 minutes
Servings: 2

Ingredients:

- ½ cup tempeh, cubed
- 1 tbsp olive oil
- 1 small zucchini, diced
- ½ cup cherry tomatoes, halved
- ½ red bell pepper, diced
- 1 medium sweet potato, peeled and cubed
- Salt and pepper, to taste
- 1 cup cooked quinoa or brown rice
- 1 tbsp tahini
- 1 tbsp lemon juice
- Water, to thin dressing

Instructions:

1. Preheat oven to 400°F (200°C). Line a baking sheet with parchment paper.

2. Place the tempeh, zucchini, cherry tomatoes, bell pepper, and sweet potato on the baking sheet. Drizzle with olive oil, season with salt and pepper, and toss to coat.

3. Roast for 20-25 minutes, stirring halfway through, until the veggies are tender and the tempeh is lightly golden.

4. In a small bowl, whisk together the tahini, lemon juice, and enough water to create a drizzling consistency.

5. Divide the cooked quinoa or brown rice into bowls and top with the roasted veggies and tempeh.

6. Drizzle with the tahini dressing and serve warm.

Nutritional Values (per serving):
- **Calories**: ~350 kcal
- **Protein**: 14g
- **Carbohydrates**: 50g
- **Fiber**: 8g
- **Sugars**: 7g
- **Fat**: 12g

Cucumber Avocado Rice Sushi Rolls

Prep Time: 15 minutes
Cook Time: 20 minutes (for rice)
Servings: 2 (makes approximately 4 rolls)

Ingredients:
- 1 cup sushi rice
- 1¼ cups water (for cooking rice)
- 1 tbsp rice vinegar
- ½ tsp sugar
- ¼ tsp salt
- 1 medium cucumber, julienned
- ½ ripe avocado, sliced thinly
- 4 sheets nori (seaweed)
- Soy sauce or tamari (low-sodium, for dipping)
- Pickled ginger (optional, for garnish)

Instructions:
1. Rinse the sushi rice under cold water until the water runs clear. Place the rice and water in a small pot and bring to a boil. Reduce heat to low, cover, and simmer for 15 minutes. Remove from heat and let it sit, covered, for another 10 minutes.

2. In a small bowl, mix the rice vinegar, sugar, and salt. Gently fold this mixture into the cooked rice until it's evenly coated. Let the rice cool to room temperature.

3. **Assemble the Rolls**: Place one sheet of nori on a bamboo sushi mat (or clean surface) with the shiny side down. Wet your hands slightly to prevent sticking, and spread a thin, even layer of rice over the nori, leaving a 1-inch border at the top edge.

4. Place a few strips of cucumber and avocado along the center of the rice.

5. Using the bamboo mat, carefully roll the sushi away from you, pressing gently to form a tight roll. Seal the edge with a bit of water if needed.

6. Repeat with the remaining ingredients.

7. Slice each roll into bite-sized pieces with a sharp, damp knife.

8. Serve with low-sodium soy sauce or tamari and pickled ginger on the side.

Nutritional Values (per serving):

- **Calories**: ~250 kcal; **Protein**: 4g
- **Carbohydrates**: 45g; **Fiber**: 4g
- **Fat**: 6g

CHAPTER 6

DINNER RECIPES

Stir-Fried Tofu with Zucchini and Carrots

Prep Time: 10 minutes
Cook Time: 15 minutes
Servings: 2

Ingredients:

- 1 tbsp sesame oil or olive oil
- ½ cup firm tofu, cubed
- 1 medium zucchini, sliced
- 1 medium carrot, julienned
- 1 tbsp low-sodium tamari or soy sauce
- 1 tsp fresh ginger, grated (or ¼ tsp ground ginger)
- Salt and pepper, to taste
- Fresh cilantro or green onion tops, for garnish (optional)

Instructions:

1. Heat oil in a skillet over medium heat. Add tofu cubes and cook until golden on all sides, about 5-6 minutes. Remove tofu from skillet and set aside.

2. In the same skillet, add zucchini and carrots. Stir-fry for 4-5 minutes until vegetables are tender-crisp.

3. Add the tofu back to the skillet. Add tamari or soy sauce, and grated ginger. Stir well and cook for another 2-3 minutes to combine flavors.

4. Season with salt and pepper to taste, and garnish with cilantro or green onion tops if desired.

5. Serve warm.

Nutritional Val (per serving):

- **Calories**: ~180 kcal; **Protein**: 9g
- **Carbohydrates**: 12g
- **Fiber**: 4g
- **Sugars**: 3g
- **Fat**: 10g

Stuffed Sweet Potatoes with Spinach and Quinoa

Prep Time: 10 minutes
Cook Time: 45 minutes
Servings: 2

Ingredients:

- 2 medium sweet potatoes
- ½ cup cooked quinoa
- 1 cup fresh spinach, chopped
- 1 tbsp olive oil
- Salt and pepper, to taste
- 1 tbsp tahini
- 1 tbsp lemon juice
- Fresh parsley, for garnish (optional)

Instructions:

1. Preheat oven to 400°F (200°C). Wash and dry the sweet potatoes, then pierce them with a fork. Place on a baking sheet and roast for 40-45 minutes, until tender.

2. While the sweet potatoes are baking, prepare the quinoa according to package instructions if not already cooked.

3. In a skillet, heat olive oil over medium heat. Add spinach and cook until wilted, about 2-3 minutes. Season with salt and pepper.

4. In a small bowl, mix the tahini and lemon juice, adding a bit of water if needed to reach a drizzling consistency.

5. Once the sweet potatoes are cooked, slice them open and fluff the insides with a fork. Fill each sweet potato with cooked quinoa and spinach.

6. Drizzle with the tahini-lemon sauce and garnish with parsley if desired. Serve warm.

Nutritional Values (per serving):
- **Calories**: ~300 kcal
- **Protein**: 7g
- **Carbohydrates**: 55g
- **Fiber**: 7g
- **Sugars**: 9g
- **Fat**: 8g

Roasted Vegetable and Brown Rice Bowl

Prep Time: 15 minutes
Cook Time: 30 minutes
Servings: 2

Ingredients:

- 1 cup cooked brown rice
- ½ cup cherry tomatoes, halved
- 1 medium zucchini, sliced
- ½ red bell pepper, diced
- 1 medium carrot, sliced
- 1 tbsp olive oil
- Salt and pepper, to taste
- 1 tbsp tahini
- 1 tbsp apple cider vinegar
- Water, to thin dressing
- Fresh parsley or cilantro, for garnish (optional)

Instructions:

1. Preheat oven to 400°F (200°C). Line a baking sheet with parchment paper.

2. Arrange the cherry tomatoes, zucchini, bell pepper, and carrot on the baking sheet. Drizzle with olive oil, and season with salt and pepper. Toss to coat.

3. Roast for 25-30 minutes, or until vegetables are tender and slightly caramelized.

4. In a small bowl, mix tahini and apple cider vinegar. Add water a little at a time until the dressing reaches a drizzling consistency.

5. To assemble, divide the cooked brown rice between two bowls. Top with roasted vegetables and drizzle with the tahini dressing.

6. Garnish with fresh parsley or cilantro if desired and serve warm.

Nutritional Values (per serving):

- **Calories**: ~350 kcal
- **Protein**: 8g
- **Carbohydrates**: 60g
- **Fiber**: 8g
- **Sugars**: 6g
- **Fat**: 12g

Tempeh Tacos with Cabbage and Lime Slaw

Prep Time: 15 minutes
Cook Time: 10 minutes
Servings: 2 (makes 4 tacos)

Ingredients:

For the Tempeh:

- ½ cup tempeh, crumbled
- 1 tbsp olive oil
- ½ tsp ground cumin
- ½ tsp smoked paprika
- Salt and pepper, to taste

For the Slaw:

- 1 cup red or green cabbage, thinly sliced
- 1 tbsp lime juice
- 1 tsp olive oil
- Salt, to taste

For the Tacos:

- 4 small corn tortillas
- Fresh cilantro, for garnish (optional)

Instructions:

1. **Prepare the Tempeh**: In a skillet, heat olive oil over medium heat. Add the crumbled tempeh, cumin, smoked paprika, salt, and pepper. Sauté for 5-7 minutes, until the tempeh is golden and fragrant.

2. **Make the Slaw**: In a small bowl, combine the cabbage, lime juice, olive oil, and a pinch of salt. Toss well to coat and let sit for 5 minutes to allow the flavors to meld.

3. **Assemble the Tacos**: Warm the corn tortillas in a dry skillet or microwave. Divide the tempeh mixture evenly among the tortillas. Top with the cabbage slaw and garnish with fresh cilantro if desired.

4. Serve warm.

Nutritional Val (per serving):

- **Calories**: ~250 kcal; **Protein**: 8g
- **Carbohydrates**: 32g; **Fiber**: 6g
- **Sugars**: 2g
- **Fat**: 10g

Coconut Curry with Bell Peppers and Carrots

Prep Time: 10 minutes
Cook Time: 20 minutes
Servings: 2

Ingredients:

- 1 tbsp coconut oil
- 1 small red bell pepper, sliced
- 1 medium carrot, julienned
- 1 cup canned coconut milk (full-fat or light)
- 1 tsp ground turmeric
- ½ tsp ground ginger (or 1 tsp fresh grated ginger)
- 1 tbsp lime juice
- Salt and pepper, to taste
- Fresh basil or cilantro, for garnish (optional)

Instructions:

1. In a medium pot, heat coconut oil over medium heat. Add the bell pepper and carrot, and sauté for 5 minutes until they begin to soften.

2. Add the coconut milk, turmeric, and ginger. Stir well and bring to a gentle simmer. Reduce heat and cook for 10-12 minutes, or until the vegetables are tender.

3. Add lime juice and season with salt and pepper to taste.

4. Serve warm, garnished with fresh basil or cilantro if desired.

Nutritional Values (per serving):

- **Calories**: ~280 kcal
- **Protein**: 3g
- **Carbohydrates**: 10g
- **Fiber**: 4g
- **Sugars**: 3g
- **Fat**: 26g

Eggplant and Tomato Stew with Fresh Herbs

Prep Time: 10 minutes
Cook Time: 30 minutes
Servings: 2

Ingredients:

- 1 tbsp olive oil
- 1 medium eggplant, diced
- 1 cup diced tomatoes (fresh or canned, no added garlic or onions)
- ½ cup vegetable broth
- 1 tsp dried oregano
- 1 tsp dried basil
- Salt and pepper, to taste
- Fresh parsley, for garnish (optional)

Instructions:

1. In a medium pot, heat olive oil over medium heat. Add the diced eggplant and cook for 5-7 minutes, stirring occasionally, until it starts to soften.

2. Add the tomatoes, vegetable broth, oregano, and basil. Stir well, cover, and let simmer for 20-25 minutes, until the eggplant is tender and the flavors have melded.

3. Season with salt and pepper to taste.

4. Serve warm, garnished with fresh parsley if desired.

Nutritional Values (per serving):
- **Calories**: ~150 kcal
- **Protein**: 3g
- **Carbohydrates**: 20g
- **Fiber**: 6g
- **Sugars**: 7g
- **Fat**: 7g

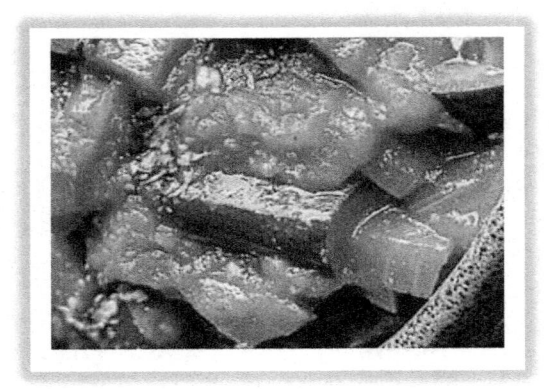

Baked Spaghetti Squash

Prep Time: 10 minutes
Cook Time: 45 minutes
Servings: 2

Ingredients:

- 1 medium spaghetti squash
- 1 tbsp olive oil
- Salt and pepper, to taste
- 1½ cups marinara sauce (ensure it is free from garlic and onion)
- 1 cup fresh spinach, chopped
- Fresh basil, for garnish (optional)

Instructions:

1. Preheat the oven to 400°F (200°C). Cut the spaghetti squash in half lengthwise and remove the seeds. Drizzle the inside with olive oil, and season with salt and pepper.

2. Place the squash halves, cut-side down, on a baking sheet and roast for 35-45 minutes, or until the flesh is tender and easily shreds into spaghetti-like strands with a fork.

3. While the squash bakes, heat the marinara sauce in a saucepan over low heat. Once heated, add the chopped spinach and cook until wilted, about 3-4 minutes.

4. Once the squash is done, use a fork to scrape the flesh into spaghetti-like strands. Spoon the marinara and spinach mixture over the top.

5. Garnish with fresh basil and serve warm.

Nutritional Values (per serving):

- **Calories**: ~220 kcal
- **Protein**: 6g
- **Carbohydrates**: 35g
- **Fiber**: 7g
- **Sugars**: 8g
- **Fat**: 7g

Ginger and Turmeric Lentil Soup

Prep Time: 10 minutes
Cook Time: 20 minutes
Servings: 2

Ingredients:

- 1 tbsp olive oil
- 1 tsp fresh ginger, grated (or ½ tsp ground ginger)
- 1 tsp ground turmeric
- 2 cups vegetable broth (low-sodium)
- 1 can (15 oz) lentils, drained and rinsed
- Salt and pepper, to taste
- 1 tbsp fresh lemon juice
- Fresh cilantro, for garnish (optional)

Instructions:

1. In a medium pot, heat olive oil over medium heat. Add the grated ginger and ground turmeric, and sauté for 1-2 minutes until fragrant.
2. Add the vegetable broth and bring to a simmer.

3. Stir in the rinsed lentils, season with salt and pepper, and let the soup simmer for 10-15 minutes, allowing the flavors to meld together.

4. Remove from heat and stir in the lemon juice.

5. Serve warm, garnished with fresh cilantro if desired.

Nutritional Values (per serving):
- **Calories**: ~250 kcal
- **Protein**: 12g
- **Carbohydrates**: 40g
- **Fiber**: 12g
- **Sugars**: 4g
- **Fat**: 4g

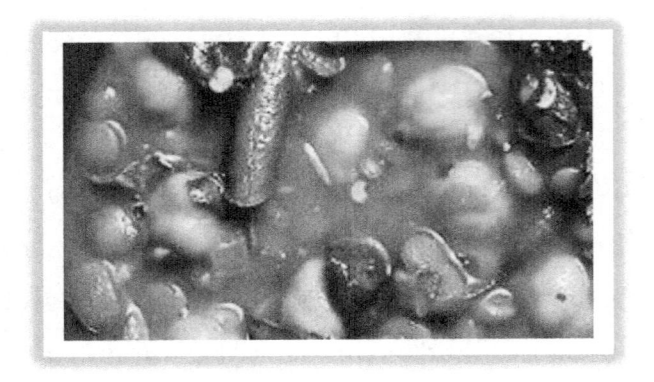

Baked Polenta with Tomato Sauce

Prep Time: 10 minutes
Cook Time: 40 minutes
Servings: 2

Ingredients:

- 1 package (about 12 oz) pre-cooked polenta, sliced into ½-inch rounds
- 1 tbsp olive oil
- Salt and pepper, to taste
- 1 cup zucchini, sliced
- 1 red bell pepper, sliced
- 1 cup cherry tomatoes, halved
- 1 cup tomato sauce (ensure it is free from garlic and onion)
- Fresh basil, for garnish (optional)

Instructions:

1. Preheat the oven to 400°F (200°C). Place the sliced polenta rounds on a baking sheet, drizzle with olive oil, and season with salt and pepper.

Bake for 15-20 minutes, flipping halfway through, until golden and crispy.

2. While the polenta bakes, arrange the zucchini, bell pepper, and cherry tomatoes on another baking sheet. Drizzle with olive oil, season with salt and pepper, and roast for 20-25 minutes, or until tender and slightly caramelized.

3. While the vegetables are roasting, heat the tomato sauce in a saucepan over low heat.

4. Once everything is ready, arrange the baked polenta rounds on a plate, top with roasted vegetables, and drizzle with tomato sauce.

5. Garnish with fresh basil and serve warm.

Nutritional Values (per serving):

- **Calories**: ~300 kcal
- **Protein**: 7g
- **Carbohydrates**: 50g
- **Fiber**: 9g
- **Sugars**: 12g
- **Fat**: 10g

CHAPTER 7

SOUPS AND STEWS

Creamy Carrot Ginger Soup

Prep Time: 10 minutes
Cook Time: 20 minutes
Servings: 2

Ingredients:

- 1 tbsp olive oil
- 4 medium carrots, chopped
- 1 tsp fresh ginger, grated (or ½ tsp ground ginger)
- 2 cups low-sodium vegetable broth
- ½ cup canned coconut milk
- Salt and pepper, to taste
- Fresh parsley, for garnish (optional)

Instructions:

1. Heat olive oil in a medium pot over medium heat. Add the carrots and ginger, and sauté for 5 minutes until softened.

2. Add vegetable broth, bring to a boil, then reduce heat to simmer. Cook for 15 minutes, or until carrots are tender.

3. Remove from heat. Use an immersion blender or transfer to a blender to blend until smooth.

4. Stir in the coconut milk, and season with salt and pepper to taste.

5. Serve warm, garnished with fresh parsley if desired.

Nutritional Values (per serving):
- **Calories**: ~150 kcal
- **Protein**: 2g
- **Carbohydrates**: 18g
- **Fiber**: 4g
- **Sugars**: 7g
- **Fat**: 8g

Roasted Red Pepper Tomato Soup

Prep Time: 10 minutes
Cook Time: 25 minutes
Servings: 2

Ingredients:

- 1 tbsp olive oil
- 1 large red bell pepper, roasted and peeled
- 1 cup diced tomatoes (canned, no garlic or onions added)
- 1½ cups low-sodium vegetable broth
- 1 tsp apple cider vinegar
- Salt and pepper, to taste
- Fresh basil leaves, for garnish (optional)

Instructions:

1. In a medium pot, heat olive oil over medium heat. Add the diced tomatoes and roasted red pepper. Sauté for 5 minutes until softened.

2. Add vegetable broth and bring to a boil. Reduce heat and let it simmer for 15-20 minutes.

3. Remove from heat and use an immersion blender (or transfer to a blender) to blend until smooth.

4. Stir in the apple cider vinegar and season with salt and pepper to taste.

5. Serve warm, garnished with fresh basil leaves if desired.

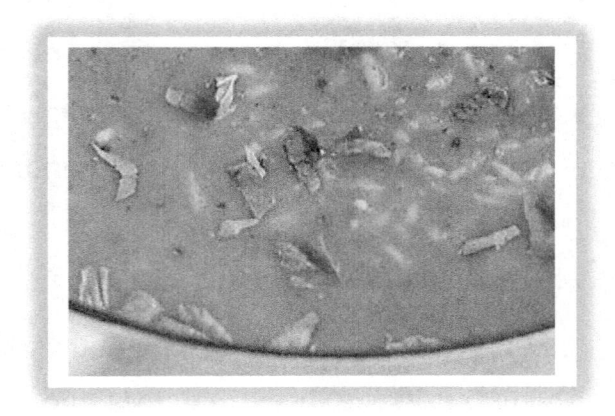

Butternut Squash Sage Soup

Prep Time: 10 minutes
Cook Time: 30 minutes
Servings: 4

Ingredients:

- 1 tbsp olive oil
- 1 medium butternut squash, peeled and cubed
- 1 medium carrot, sliced
- 1 tsp fresh sage, chopped (or ½ tsp dried sage)
- 4 cups low-sodium vegetable broth
- Salt and pepper, to taste
- Fresh parsley, for garnish (optional)

Instructions:

1. In a large pot, heat olive oil over medium heat. Add butternut squash and carrot, and sauté for 5 minutes, until they start to soften.

2. Add the sage and stir for about 1 minute until fragrant.

3. Pour in the vegetable broth and bring to a boil. Reduce heat, cover, and let simmer for 20 minutes or until the squash and carrot are tender.

4. Using an immersion blender (or carefully in a regular blender in batches), blend the soup until smooth.

5. Season with salt and pepper to taste and garnish with fresh parsley if desired.

6. Serve warm.

Nutritional Val. (per serving):

- **Calories**: ~130 kcal
- **Protein**: 2g
- **Carbohydrates**: 24g
- **Fiber**: 4g
- **Sugars**: 5g
- **Fat**: 4g

Pumpkin Bell Pepper Stew

Prep Time: 10 minutes
Cook Time: 25 minutes
Servings: 4

Ingredients:

- 1 tbsp coconut oil or olive oil
- 1 cup canned pumpkin puree (unsweetened)
- 1 red bell pepper, diced
- 1 yellow bell pepper, diced
- ½ tsp ground turmeric
- ½ tsp ground cumin
- 3 cups low-sodium vegetable broth
- Salt and pepper, to taste
- Fresh cilantro, for garnish (optional)

Instructions:

1. In a large pot, heat coconut oil over medium heat. Add the bell peppers and sauté for 5 minutes until they soften slightly.

2. Add the pumpkin puree, turmeric, and cumin. Stir well to combine.

3. Pour in the vegetable broth, bring to a simmer, and cook for 15-20 minutes until the stew thickens and flavors meld.

4. Season with salt and pepper to taste and garnish with fresh cilantro if desired.

5. Serve warm.

Nutritional Values (per serving):

- **Calories**: ~120 kcal
- **Protein**: 3g
- **Carbohydrates**: 18g
- **Fiber**: 4g
- **Sugars**: 7g
- **Fat**: 4g

Zucchini and Corn Chowder

Prep Time: 10 minutes
Cook Time: 20 minutes
Servings: 4

Ingredients

- 1 tbsp olive oil
- 1 medium zucchini, diced
- 1 cup canned corn kernels, drained and rinsed
- 1 medium carrot, diced
- 1 stalk green onion (green tops only), chopped
- 1 medium potato, peeled and diced
- 3 cups low-sodium vegetable broth
- ½ cup lactose-free milk or unsweetened almond milk
- Salt and pepper, to taste
- Fresh parsley, chopped, for garnish

Instructions

1. In a large pot, heat olive oil over medium heat. Add zucchini, carrot, green onion tops, and potato. Sauté for 5 minutes, until vegetables are slightly softened.

2. Add the vegetable broth and bring to a boil. Reduce heat and let simmer for 15 minutes, or until the vegetables are tender.

3. Add the corn and lactose-free milk (or almond milk) to the pot. Stir well and cook for an additional 2-3 minutes to heat through.

4. Season with salt and pepper to taste. Garnish with fresh parsley before serving.

Nutritional Info (per serving)
- **Calories**: 120 kcal
- **Protein**: 3 g
- **Carbohydrates**: 20 g
- **Fiber**: 4 g
- **Sugars**: 4 g
- **Fat**: 4 g
- **Saturated Fat**: 0.5 g
- **Calcium**: 60 mg
- **Iron**: 1 mg

Sweet Potato and Coconut Milk Stew

Prep Time: 10 minutes
Cook Time: 25 minutes
Servings: 4

Nutritional Val. (per serving):
Calories: ~200 kcal; Protein: 2g
Carbs: 23g; Fiber: 4g; Fat: 10g

Ingredients:
- 1 tbsp olive oil
- 1 medium sweet potato, peeled and cubed
- 1 medium zucchini, diced
- 1 cup canned coconut milk (full-fat or light)
- 2 cups low-sodium vegetable broth
- ½ tsp ground ginger
- Salt and pepper, to taste
- Fresh basil, for garnish (optional)

Instructions:
1. In a large pot, heat olive oil over medium heat. Add the sweet potato and sauté for 5 minutes.

2. Add the zucchini, coconut milk, vegetable broth, and ground ginger. Stir well and bring to a simmer.

3. Cook for 15-20 minutes, or until the sweet potato is tender and the stew has thickened.

4. Season with salt and pepper to taste and garnish with fresh basil if desired.

5. Serve warm.

Spinach Potato Dill Soup

Prep Time: 10 minutes
Cook Time: 20 minutes
Servings: 4

Nutritional Info (per serving)
Calories: 130 kcal; Protein: 3 g
Carbs: 20 g; Fiber: 4 g;
Fat: 4 g; Saturated Fat: 0.5 g

Ingredients

- 1 tbsp olive oil
- 2 medium potatoes, peeled and diced
- 3 cups low-sodium vegetable broth
- 3 cups fresh spinach, chopped
- 1 tbsp fresh dill, chopped
- Salt and pepper, to taste

Instructions

1. Heat olive oil in a large pot over medium heat. Add diced potatoes and cook, stirring for about 5 minutes.

2. Pour in the vegetable broth and bring to a boil. Reduce heat and simmer for 10-15 minutes, or until potatoes are tender.

3. Add spinach and cook for an additional 2 minutes, until spinach is wilted.

4. Stir in fresh dill, season with salt and pepper, and serve warm.

Celeriac Parsnip Soup

Prep Time: 10 minutes
Cook Time: 25 minutes
Servings: 4

Ingredients:

- 1 tbsp olive oil
- 1 medium celeriac (celery root), peeled and diced
- 2 medium parsnips, peeled and diced
- 1 small carrot, sliced
- 4 cups low-sodium vegetable broth
- 1 tsp fresh thyme (or ½ tsp dried thyme)
- Salt and pepper, to taste
- Fresh parsley, for garnish (optional)

Instructions:

1. In a large pot, heat olive oil over medium heat. Add the celeriac, parsnips, and carrot, and sauté for 5 minutes, stirring occasionally.

2. Add the vegetable broth and thyme. Bring to a boil, then reduce heat and simmer for 20 minutes, until vegetables are tender.

3. Using an immersion blender (or carefully in a regular blender), blend until smooth.

4. Season with salt and pepper to taste and garnish with fresh parsley if desired.

5. Serve warm.

Nutritional Values (per serving):

- **Calories**: ~100 kcal
- **Protein**: 2g
- **Carbohydrates**: 18g
- **Fiber**: 5g
- **Sugars**: 5g
- **Fat**: 3g

Spinach and Quinoa Vegetable Soup

Prep Time: 10 minutes
Cook Time: 20 minutes
Servings: 4

Ingredients:

- 1 tbsp olive oil
- 1 medium carrot, sliced
- 1 small zucchini, diced
- 1 cup fresh spinach
- ¼ cup quinoa, rinsed
- 4 cups low-sodium vegetable broth
- 1 tsp fresh basil, chopped (or ½ tsp dried basil)
- Salt and pepper, to taste

Instructions:

1. In a large pot, heat olive oil over medium heat. Add the carrot and zucchini and sauté for 5 minutes, until they begin to soften.

2. Add the vegetable broth and quinoa. Bring to a boil, then reduce heat and simmer for 15 minutes, until the quinoa is cooked and the vegetables are tender.

3. Stir in the spinach and cook for an additional 2-3 minutes, until wilted.

4. Season with basil, salt, and pepper to taste.

5. Serve warm.

Nutritional Values (per serving):
- **Calories**: ~120 kcal
- **Protein**: 4g
- **Carbohydrates**: 16g
- **Fiber**: 3g
- **Sugars**: 3g
- **Fat**: 4g

CHAPTER 8

SNACKS AND DESSERTS

Almond Butter Chia Energy Balls

Prep Time: 10 minutes
Chill Time: 30 minutes
Servings: 12 balls

Ingredients:

- 1 cup rolled oats (certified gluten-free if necessary)
- ¼ cup almond butter
- 2 tbsp shredded unsweetened coconut
- 1 tbsp chia seeds
- 2 tbsp maple syrup
- ¼ tsp cinnamon (optional)
- A pinch of salt

Instructions:

1. In a medium bowl, combine the oats, almond butter, shredded coconut, chia seeds, maple syrup, cinnamon, and salt. Stir until well mixed.
2. Using your hands, roll the mixture into small balls, about 1 inch in diameter.
3. Place the balls on a tray and refrigerate for at least 30 minutes to firm up.
4. Store in an airtight container in the fridge for up to a week.

Nutritional Values (per energy ball):

- **Calories**: ~80 kcal
- **Protein**: 2g
- **Carbohydrates**: 9g
- **Fiber**: 1g
- **Sugars**: 3g
- **Fat**: 4g

Blueberry Chia Pudding Parfait

Prep Time: 5 minutes
Chill Time: 4 hours or overnight
Servings: 2

Ingredients:

- 1 cup unsweetened almond milk
- 3 tbsp chia seeds
- 1 tbsp maple syrup
- ¼ cup fresh blueberries
- 2 tbsp shredded unsweetened coconut (optional)

Instructions:

1. In a medium bowl or mason jar, mix the almond milk, chia seeds, and maple syrup. Stir well to combine.

2. Cover and refrigerate for at least 4 hours or overnight, stirring once after an hour to prevent clumping.

3. Once the chia pudding has set, layer it in serving glasses with fresh blueberries and shredded coconut.

4. Serve chilled.

Lemon Coconut Energy Balls

Prep Time: 10 minutes
Servings: 8 energy balls

Ingredients

- 1 cup unsweetened shredded coconut
- 1 tbsp lemon zest (from about 1 lemon)
- 2 tbsp pure maple syrup
- 1 tbsp coconut oil, melted
- ¼ tsp vanilla extract
- Pinch of salt

Instructions

1. In a food processor, pulse the shredded coconut, lemon zest, maple syrup, coconut oil, vanilla, and salt until the mixture sticks together.

2. Scoop about 1 tablespoon of the mixture, roll into a ball, and place on a plate.

3. Repeat with the remaining mixture to make 8 balls.

4. Refrigerate for 15 minutes to firm up before serving.

Nutritional Info (per energy ball)
- **Calories**: 70 kcal; **Protein**: 1 g; **Carbs**: 4 g
- **Fiber**: 2 g; **Calcium**: 5 mg; **Iron**: 0.2 mg

Banana and Oatmeal Cookies

Prep Time: 5 minutes
Cook Time: 12 minutes
Servings: 10 cookies

Ingredients:
- 1 ripe banana, mashed
- 1 cup rolled oats (certified gluten-free if necessary)
- 2 tbsp almond butter
- 1 tbsp maple syrup
- ¼ tsp cinnamon
- ¼ cup unsweetened shredded coconut (optional)

Instructions:
1. Preheat your oven to 350°F (175°C) and line a baking sheet with parchment paper.
2. In a medium bowl, combine the mashed banana, oats, almond butter, maple syrup, and cinnamon. Mix until well combined.

3. Drop spoonfuls of the mixture onto the prepared baking sheet and press down gently to flatten each cookie slightly.

4. Bake for 10-12 minutes or until the cookies are golden brown.

5. Allow to cool on the baking sheet for a few minutes, then transfer to a wire rack to cool completely.

Nutritional Values (per cookie):
- **Calories**: ~70 kcal
- **Protein**: 1g
- **Carbohydrates**: 10g
- **Fiber**: 2g
- **Sugars**: 3g
- **Fat**: 2g

Cinnamon Roasted Pumpkin Seeds

Prep Time: 5 minutes
Cook Time: 15 minutes
Servings: 4

Nutritional Val. (per serving):
Calories: ~100 kcal; Protein: 3g
Carbs: 4g; Fiber: 1g; Fat: 9g

Ingredients:
- 1 cup raw pumpkin seeds
- 1 tbsp coconut oil, melted
- 1 tsp cinnamon
- 1 tsp maple syrup
- A pinch of salt

Instructions:
1. Preheat your oven to 350°F (175°C) and line a baking sheet with parchment paper.

2. In a bowl, combine the pumpkin seeds, melted coconut oil, cinnamon, maple syrup, and salt. Mix until the seeds are well coated.

3. Spread the pumpkin seeds in a single layer on the prepared baking sheet.

4. Bake for 12-15 minutes, stirring halfway through, until the seeds are golden and crisp.

5. Allow the seeds to cool completely before serving or storing in an airtight container.

Coconut Yogurt with Kiwi and Strawberries

Prep Time: 5 minutes
Servings: 1

Ingredients:

- 1 cup unsweetened coconut yogurt
- 1 kiwi, peeled and sliced
- 2-3 strawberries, sliced
- 1 tbsp chia seeds (optional)

Instructions:

1. Place the coconut yogurt in a serving bowl.

2. Top with sliced kiwi, strawberries, and chia seeds if desired.

3. Serve immediately or refrigerate for later.

Nutritional Values (per serving):

- **Calories:** ~150 kcal
- **Protein:** 2g
- **Carbohydrates:** 15g
- **Fiber:** 5g
- **Sugars:** 7g
- **Fat:** 9g

Chocolate-Dipped Rice Cakes with Almonds

Prep Time: 10 minutes
Cook Time: 5 minutes
Servings: 6 rice cakes

Ingredients:

- 6 plain rice cakes (check for low-FODMAP, no added ingredients)
- ⅓ cup dark chocolate chips (dairy-free, 70% or higher)
- 2 tbsp almond slivers
- 1 tsp coconut oil

Instructions:

1. In a microwave-safe bowl, combine the dark chocolate chips and coconut oil. Microwave in 20-second intervals, stirring each time until smooth and melted.

2. Dip half of each rice cake into the melted chocolate, letting excess drip off.

3. Place the dipped rice cakes on a parchment-lined baking sheet.

4. Sprinkle with almond slivers while the chocolate is still warm.

5. Refrigerate for 10 minutes, or until the chocolate is set.

6. Serve or store in an airtight container in the fridge.

Nutritional Values (per rice cake):
- **Calories**: ~100 kcal
- **Protein**: 1g
- **Carbohydrates**: 12g
- **Fiber**: 1g
- **Sugars**: 3g
- **Fat**: 5g

Peanut Butter Banana Nice Cream

Prep Time: 5 minutes

Servings: 2

Ingredients:

- 2 ripe bananas, sliced and frozen
- 1 tbsp natural peanut butter (ensure it's smooth and unsweetened)
- ¼ tsp vanilla extract (optional)

Instructions:

1. Place the frozen banana slices in a high-speed blender or food processor.
2. Blend until smooth and creamy, stopping to scrape down the sides as needed.
3. Add the peanut butter and vanilla extract (if using) and blend until well combined.
4. Serve immediately for a soft-serve texture or freeze for an additional 30 minutes if you prefer a firmer consistency.

Nutritional Values (per serving):

- **Calories**: ~150 kcal; **Protein**: 3g
- **Carbs**: 30g; **Fiber**: 4g; **Fat**: 4g

Baked Carrot Chips with Paprika

Prep Time: 5 minutes
Cook Time: 20 minutes
Servings: 2

Ingredients:
- 2 large carrots, peeled and thinly sliced (about 1/8-inch thick)
- 1 tsp olive oil
- ½ tsp smoked paprika (or regular paprika if preferred)
- Salt, to taste
- Black pepper, to taste (optional)

Instructions:
1. Preheat your oven to 400°F (200°C) and line a baking sheet with parchment paper.

2. In a mixing bowl, toss the carrot slices with olive oil, paprika, salt, and pepper (if using) until evenly coated.

3. Arrange the carrot slices in a single layer on the prepared baking sheet.

4. Bake for 15-20 minutes, flipping halfway through, until the chips are crispy and golden brown. Watch carefully to prevent burning.

5. Allow to cool slightly before serving.

CHAPTER 9

SMOOTHIES AND BEVERAGES

Peach and Ginger Smoothie

Prep Time: 5 minutes
Servings: 1

Ingredients

- 1 medium ripe peach, pitted and sliced
- ½ inch fresh ginger, peeled and grated
- ½ cup unsweetened almond milk
- ½ cup ice cubes
- 1 tbsp chia seeds (optional)

Instructions

1. In a blender, combine the sliced peach, grated ginger, almond milk, ice cubes, and chia seeds (if using).

2. Blend until smooth and creamy.

3. Serve immediately in a glass.

Blueberry and Coconut Water Smoothie

Prep Time: 5 minutes
Servings: 1

Ingredients:

- 1 cup coconut water (unsweetened)
- ½ cup fresh or frozen blueberries
- ¼ cup baby spinach (optional for added greens)
- 1 tbsp chia seeds
- Ice cubes, as needed

Instructions:

1. In a blender, add coconut water, blueberries, baby spinach (if using), and chia seeds.
2. Blend on high until smooth, adding ice cubes for a thicker texture if desired.
3. Pour into a glass and enjoy immediately.

Nutritional Values (per serving):

- **Calories**: ~90 kcal; **Protein**: 2g
- **Carbs**: 20g; **Fiber**: 4g
- **Sugars**: 12g
- **Fat**: 1g

Pineapple and Ginger Green Smoothie

Prep Time: 5 minutes
Servings: 1

Ingredients:

- ½ cup fresh or frozen pineapple chunks
- 1 cup unsweetened almond milk
- ½ tsp fresh ginger, grated
- ¼ cup baby spinach
- Ice cubes, as needed

Instructions:

1. In a blender, combine the pineapple, almond milk, ginger, spinach, and ice cubes.
2. Blend until smooth, adding more ice if desired for a thicker consistency.
3. Pour into a glass and enjoy immediately.

Nutritional Values (per serving):

- **Calories**: ~70 kcal; **Protein**: 1g
- **Carbohydrates**: 12g
- **Fiber**: 2g; **Sugars**: 7g
- **Fat**: 2g

Strawberry and Mint Lemonade

Prep Time: 5 minutes
Servings: 2

Ingredients:

- 1 cup fresh strawberries, hulled
- 2 cups cold water
- 1 tbsp fresh lemon juice
- 3-4 fresh mint leaves
- Ice cubes, as needed
- 1 tsp maple syrup (optional)

Instructions:

1. In a blender, combine strawberries, cold water, lemon juice, and mint leaves. Add maple syrup if desired for a hint of sweetness.
2. Blend until smooth.
3. Pour into glasses over ice and enjoy immediately.

Nutritional Val (per serving):

- **Calories**: ~25 kcal; **Protein**: 0.5g
- **Carbohydrates**: 6g
- **Fiber**: 1g

Banana and Almond Milk Smoothie

Prep Time: 5 minutes
Servings: 1

Ingredients:

- 1 medium ripe banana
- 1 cup unsweetened almond milk
- 1 tbsp almond butter
- ½ tsp vanilla extract (optional)
- Ice cubes (optional, for a thicker consistency)

Instructions:

1. In a blender, combine the banana, almond milk, almond butter, and vanilla extract (if using).
2. Blend until smooth. Add ice cubes if you prefer a colder or thicker smoothie.
3. Pour into a glass and enjoy immediately.

Nutritional Values (per serving):

- **Calories**: ~180 kcal; **Protein**: 3g
- **Carbohydrates**: 30g
- **Fiber**: 4g
- **Fat**: 6g

Turmeric Golden Milk with Coconut Milk

Prep Time: 5 minutes
Cook Time: 5 minutes
Servings: 1

Ingredients:

- 1 cup unsweetened coconut milk (from a carton)
- ½ tsp ground turmeric
- ¼ tsp ground ginger
- A pinch of black pepper (to enhance turmeric absorption)
- 1 tsp maple syrup (optional, for sweetness)

Instructions:

1. In a small saucepan, combine the coconut milk, turmeric, ginger, and black pepper.
2. Heat over medium-low heat, stirring continuously for 3-5 minutes until warm (do not boil).
3. Remove from heat, add maple syrup if desired, and stir.
4. Pour into a mug and enjoy warm.

Raspberry and Basil Infused Water

Prep Time: 5 minutes
Infuse Time: 30 minutes to 1 hour
Servings: 2

Ingredients:

- 4 cups water
- ½ cup fresh raspberries
- 4-5 fresh basil leaves

Instructions:

1. In a large pitcher, combine the water, raspberries, and basil leaves.

2. Stir gently to release some of the flavors, or muddle slightly if you prefer a stronger infusion.

3. Refrigerate for 30 minutes to 1 hour for the flavors to infuse.

4. Serve chilled and enjoy.

Nutritional Values (per serving):
- **Calories**: ~5 kcal
- **Carbohydrates**: 1g

Carrot Ginger Juice

Prep Time: 5 minutes
Servings: 2

Nutritional Val. (per serving):
Calories: ~80 kcal; Protein: 1g
Carbs: 20g; Fiber: 3g;

Ingredients:
- 2 large oranges, peeled
- 3 medium carrots, peeled
- 1-inch piece of fresh ginger, peeled
- 1 cup cold water (or coconut water for added flavor)
- Ice cubes (optional)

Instructions:

1. Place the peeled oranges, carrots, and ginger in a juicer. If you don't have a juicer, you can blend the ingredients in a blender and strain with a fine mesh sieve or cheesecloth.

2. Add cold water or coconut water to the juicer or blender to help with blending and extract the juice.

3. Blend or juice until smooth. If using a blender, strain the juice through a fine mesh sieve to remove pulp.

4. Pour the juice into glasses, add ice cubes if desired, and serve immediately.

21-DAY MEAL PLAN

Day 1
- **Breakfast**: Low-FODMAP Banana Blueberry Overnight Oats
- **Lunch**: Quinoa and Roasted Vegetable Salad
- **Dinner**: Stir-Fried Tofu with Zucchini and Carrots
- **Snack**: Almond Butter Chia Energy Balls

Day 2
- **Breakfast**: Ginger-Spiced Carrot Smoothie Bowl
- **Lunch**: Zucchini Noodle Salad with Peanut Dressing
- **Dinner**: Stuffed Sweet Potatoes with Spinach and Quinoa
- **Snack**: Blueberry Chia Pudding Parfait

Day 3
- **Breakfast**: Coconut Chia Pudding with Fresh Strawberries
- **Lunch**: Sweet Potato and Spinach Buddha Bowl
- **Dinner**: Roasted Vegetable and Brown Rice Bowl
- **Snack**: Lemon Coconut Energy Balls

Day 4
- **Breakfast**: Maple Cinnamon Quinoa Breakfast Bowl
- **Lunch**: Chickpea Salad Wraps
- **Dinner**: Tempeh Tacos with Cabbage and Lime Slaw
- **Snack**: Banana and Oatmeal Cookies

Day 5
- **Breakfast**: Spinach Bell Pepper Tofu Scramble
- **Lunch**: Mediterranean Rice Bowl
- **Dinner**: Coconut Curry with Bell Peppers and Carrots
- **Snack**: Cinnamon Roasted Pumpkin Seeds

Day 6
- **Breakfast**: Buckwheat Pancakes with Raspberries
- **Lunch**: Lentil and Bell Pepper Stuffed Bell Peppers
- **Dinner**: Eggplant and Tomato Stew with Fresh Herbs
- **Snack**: Chocolate-Dipped Rice Cakes with Almonds

Day 7
- **Breakfast**: Almond Butter and Banana Rice Cakes
- **Lunch**: Tofu and Spinach Stir-Fry with Rice Noodles
- **Dinner**: Baked Spaghetti Squash

Day 8
- **Breakfast**: Warm Oatmeal with Pumpkin Seeds and Kiwi
- **Lunch**: Carrot Ginger Soup with Coconut Milk
- **Dinner**: Ginger and Turmeric Lentil Soup
- **Snack**: Baked Carrot Chips with Paprika

Day 9
- **Breakfast**: Zucchini and Sweet Potato Hash
- **Lunch**: Tempeh and Roasted Veggie Grain Bowl
- **Dinner**: Baked Polenta with Tomato Sauce
- **Snack**: Coconut Yogurt with Kiwi and Strawberries

Day 10
- **Breakfast**: Low-FODMAP Banana Blueberry Overnight Oats
- **Lunch**: Cucumber Avocado Rice Sushi Rolls
- **Dinner**: Creamy Carrot Ginger Soup
- **Snack**: Almond Butter Chia Energy Balls

Day 11
- **Breakfast**: Ginger-Spiced Carrot Smoothie Bowl
- **Lunch**: Zucchini Noodle Salad with Peanut Dressing
- **Dinner**: Roasted Red Pepper Tomato Soup
- **Snack**: Blueberry Chia Pudding Parfait

Day 12
- **Breakfast**: Coconut Chia Pudding with Fresh Strawberries
- **Lunch**: Sweet Potato and Spinach Buddha Bowl
- **Dinner**: Butternut Squash Sage Soup
- **Snack**: Lemon Coconut Energy Balls

Day 13
- **Breakfast**: Maple Cinnamon Quinoa Breakfast Bowl
- **Lunch**: Chickpea Salad Wraps
- **Dinner**: Pumpkin Bell Pepper Stew
- **Snack**: Banana and Oatmeal Cookies

Day 14
- **Breakfast**: Spinach Bell Pepper Tofu Scramble
- **Lunch**: Mediterranean Rice Bowl
- **Dinner**: Zucchini and Corn Chowder
- **Snack**: Cinnamon Roasted Pumpkin Seeds

Day 15
- **Breakfast**: Buckwheat Pancakes with Raspberries
- **Lunch**: Lentil and Bell Pepper Stuffed Bell Peppers
- **Dinner**: Sweet Potato and Coconut Milk Stew
- **Snack**: Chocolate-Dipped Rice Cakes with Almonds

Day 16
- **Breakfast**: Almond Butter and Banana Rice Cakes
- **Lunch**: Tofu and Spinach Stir-Fry with Rice Noodles
- **Dinner**: Spinach Potato Dill Soup
- **Snack**: Peanut Butter Banana Nice Cream

Day 17
- **Breakfast**: Warm Oatmeal with Pumpkin Seeds and Kiwi
- **Lunch**: Carrot Ginger Soup with Coconut Milk
- **Dinner**: Celeriac Parsnip Soup
- **Snack**: Baked Carrot Chips with Paprika

Day 18
- **Breakfast**: Zucchini and Sweet Potato Hash
- **Lunch**: Tempeh and Roasted Veggie Grain Bowl
- **Dinner**: Spinach and Quinoa Vegetable Soup
- **Snack**: Coconut Yogurt with Kiwi and Strawberries

Day 19
- **Breakfast**: Low-FODMAP Banana Blueberry Overnight Oats
- **Lunch**: Cucumber Avocado Rice Sushi Rolls
- **Dinner**: Stir-Fried Tofu with Zucchini and Carrots
- **Snack**: Almond Butter Chia Energy Balls

Day 20
- **Breakfast**: Ginger-Spiced Carrot Smoothie Bowl
- **Lunch**: Quinoa and Roasted Vegetable Salad
- **Dinner**: Roasted Vegetable and Brown Rice Bowl
- **Snack**: Lemon Coconut Energy Balls

Day 21
- **Breakfast**: Coconut Chia Pudding with Fresh Strawberries
- **Lunch**: Sweet Potato and Spinach Buddha Bowl
- **Dinner**: Tempeh Tacos with Cabbage and Lime Slaw
- **Snack**: Banana and Oatmeal Cookies

CONCLUSION

This cookbook provides a collection of delicious, low-FODMAP recipes that cater specifically to the needs of those managing irritable bowel syndrome. Each recipe is crafted to offer satisfying meals while minimizing digestive discomfort.

Understanding your individual triggers is crucial, and this book emphasizes the importance of whole, unprocessed foods that are both nourishing and easy to prepare. From smoothies and breakfasts to hearty lunches and dinners, you'll find a variety of options that satisfy your taste buds.

As you explore these recipes, remember that everyone's experience with IBS is unique. It may take time to identify what works best for you, so listen to your body and feel free to adapt recipes to suit your tastes and tolerances.

We hope these dishes inspire you to enjoy cooking and eating while managing IBS. Thank you for allowing us to be part of your journey to better health

Happy cooking!

OTHER BOOKS BY THE AUTHOR

1. VEGAN LOW-CHOLESTEROL DIET COOKBOOK FOR SENIORS
2. THE PLANT BASED LOW-CHOLESTEROL DIET COOKBOOK FOR SENIORS
3. THE ESSENTIAL BARIATRIC DIET COOKBOOK
4. HIGH PROTEIN BARIATRIC DIET COOKBOOK FOR VEGANS
5. HIGH PROTEIN BARIATRIC DIET COOKBOOK FOR VEGETARIANS
6. VEGETARIAN ANTI-INFLAMMATORY DIET COOKBOOK FOR SENIORS
7. VEGETARIAN IRON DEFICIENCY ANEMIA COOKBOOK
8. VEGETARIAN LOW CHOLESTEROL DIET COOKBOOK FOR SENIORS
9. THE EASY DIABETIC RENAL DIET COOKBOOK FOR SENIORS
10. TYPE 2 DIABETIC AIR FRYER COOKBOOK FOR BEGINNERS
11. VEGETARIAN DIABETIC RENAL DIET COOKBOOK FOR THE NEWLY DIAGNOSED
12. THE EASY LOW SALT DIET COOKBOOK FOR SENIORS

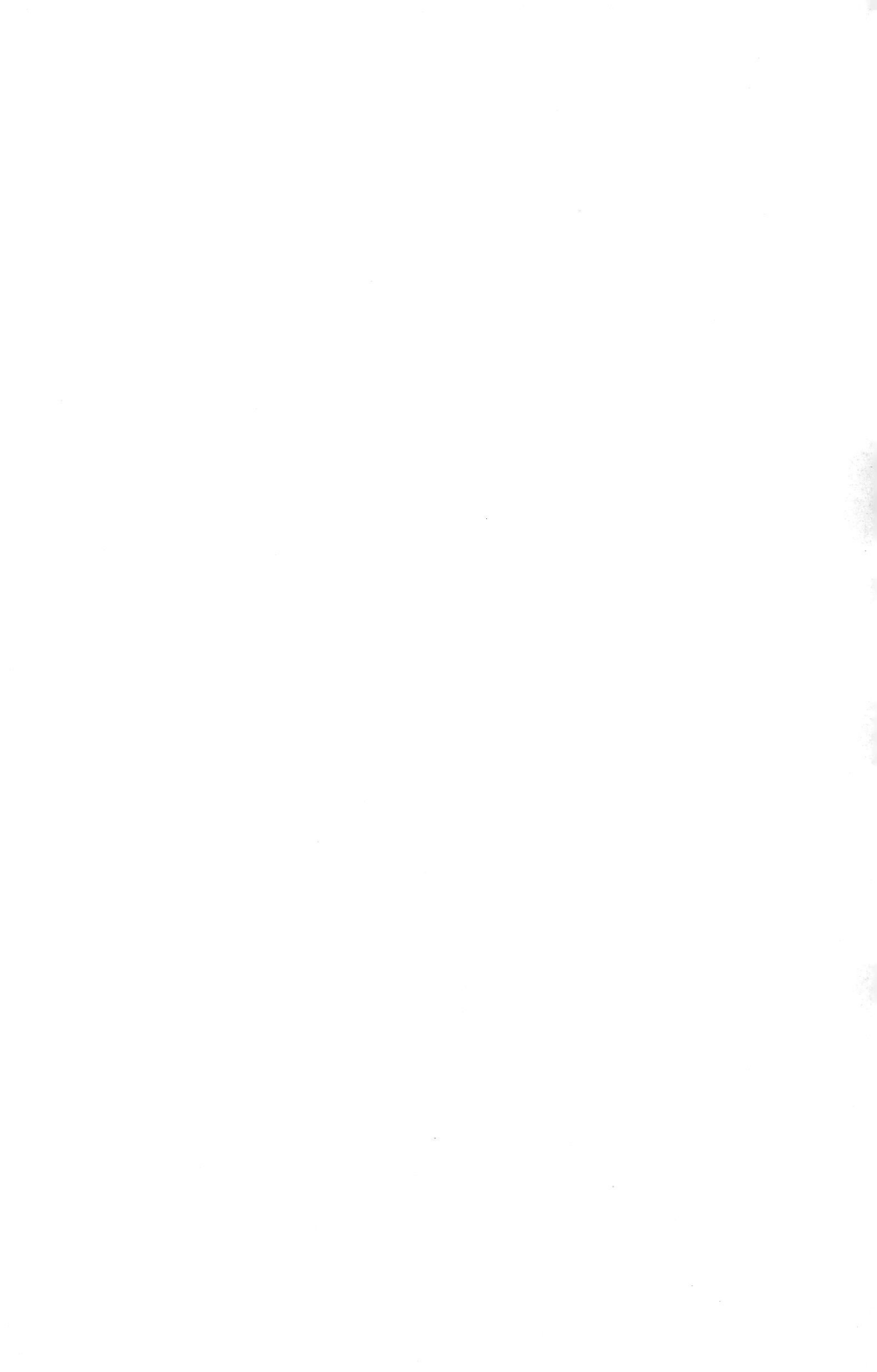

Printed in Great Britain
by Amazon